Homemade Deodorant

A Complete Beginner's Guide to

Natural DIY Deodorants You

Can Make Today

Jane Aniston

Introduction

Thank you for choosing to download *"Homemade Deodorant — A Complete Beginner's Guide to Natural DIY Deodorants You Can Make Today."*

This book contains all the information you need to know in order to start making your own natural, chemical-free deodorants at home today. The ingredients used to make these deodorants are cheap and easily available, and the process of making them couldn't be simpler!

In this book, we'll cover the differences between homemade deodorants and the store-bought variety. In addition, I'll show you why you really should ditch expensive, toxin-filled store-bought deodorants and start making your own natural, healthy, chemical-free alternatives at home.

This book also includes 20 natural deodorant recipes covering a number of various scents and deodorant types. Each recipe will list the ingredients required to make the deodorant and then guide you through the process of exactly what you'll need to do, with simple, easy-to-follow step-by-step instructions, meaning you can be making your own deodorants in no time at all!

Once you see how fantastic natural homemade deodorants are, you'll never want to go back to the harmful, store-bought variety, which can be toxic to not only your body but also the environment.

Thank you again for downloading this book. I hope you enjoy it!

Jane Aniston

Table of contents

Chapter 1: Why you should stop using store-bought deodorants and start making your own at home!

Chapter 2: Insider Tips On Creating Your Own Deodorants

Chapter 3: Fruity DIY Homemade Deodorant Recipes

1. Sweet Orange & Thyme Homemade Deodorant

2. So Citrusy Non-Toxic Deodorant

Chapter 6: Non-Toxic Oil and Butter Deodorant Recipes

Chapter 7: Mix & Match Ingredients of Natural DIY Deodorants

Chapter 1

Why you should stop using store-bought deodorant and start making your own at home!

The largest organ of the body is the skin, and one of its numerous functions is to eliminate toxins from the body. Unfortunately, it can also do the opposite, which is absorb toxins from outside of the body. For this reason, the products we choose to apply to our skin are of the utmost importance as our health can be affected by these products.

Unknown to many, the vast majority of skin care products that are commercially sold contain chemicals which are toxic to the body. The ingredients companies use to create these products can potentially cause harm to the skin instead of acting in ways which benefit it. Whats worse is that these chemical toxins can even affect our internal organs, such as the liver, kidneys and the lymphatic system. Some studies have also linked the substances used by big name manufacturers to certain cancers. Occasional use of these products is hazardous enough, but the fact that we use many of them on a daily basis makes them all the more dangerous. In this book we're going to look at store bought deodorants; a fantastic example of a product we use on a daily basis which contain some very nasty chemicals!

Deodorants are used in order to maintain dry underarms and to keep us smelling fresh throughout the day. As seen in countless commercials, deodorants help give us the confidence that comes from staying fresh and knowing that we won't smell unclean and be judged negatively by others we come into contact with. The implication is that if we don't use these products we may face social scorn.

However, perspiration is a natural function of the body which has it's uses. As well as the fact that it helps regulate our body's temperature, perspiration is actually one of the methods our body uses to detoxify.

Through it, urea, minerals, salts and fluids are removed from the body. Sweat itself is odorless, it's actually the bacteria present on the surface of our skin that is responsible for smelly underarms. When the bacteria break down compounds within the sweat, acids are formed, some of which are perceived as an unpleasant odor.

What many people are unaware of, is that commercially prepared deodorants contain parabens and aluminum. These two substances are known to be toxic to man. How? Aluminum, an ingredient which has been linked to development of breast cancer, clogs up the sweat glands to prevent them from functioning naturally, that is, it blocks the release of sweat from the body. The waste products which are usually expelled via the sweat glands are therefore kept inside the body. Furthermore, this ingredient can also accumulate and cause additional problems in the body later in life.

Parabens, on the other hand, are cosmetic, food and pharmaceutical preservatives. These compounds have been found to mimic estrogen. Although it was not officially concluded that parabens cause breast cancer, the chemical has been detected within cancerous cells gathered from malignant breast tumor biopsies. In addition, parabens supposedly affect the processes of the endocrine system. Disruption in the endocrine system can lead to problems with metabolism, growth and development, sexual function, reproduction, mood and body temperature regulation, to name just a few.

Aluminum and parabens alone pose a potential danger to our health. However, these are rarely the only harmful ingredients that can be found store bought deodorants as commercially available deodorants tend to contain a cocktail of other chemical nasties. Here are some of the other potentially harmful ingredients which regularly lurk in store-bought deodorants

- ***Propylene glycol*** - This common ingredient can cause damage to both the central nervous system and some of the body's major organs, specifically the liver and heart. Skin irritation can be initiated in those with sensitive skin, even at extremely low concentrations of the chemical. Whats more, this chemical can lead to delayed allergic reactions. Unfortunately, propylene glycol is found in many "natural" deodorants, even up to fairly high concentrations.

- **Triclosan** - According to the FDA, triclosan is actually a classified pesticide! Triclosan is used in deodorants as an antibacterial agent and preservative The problem is that triclosan destroys not only the "bad" bacteria, but also the body's "good" bacteria. Triclosan is listed as a possible carcinogen by the IARC and it is also thought that this nasty chemical disrupts endocrine function, as evidenced by the study of human blood and breast milk.

- **Steareths** - When listed as an ingredient on product packaging these nasty chemicals are usually followed by a number (e.g. steareth-15). These cheap additives are derived from vegetables but undergo a process (known as ethoxylation) which involves the known carcinogen ethylene-oxide.

- **Fragrance** – The term "fragrance" is used as a catchall for a number of chemicals which can cause skin irritation, allergies and toxicity in the organs of the body, not to mention they're harmful to the environment.

- **Talc** - Talc is thought to contain asbestiform fibers, which could make it a potential carcinogen. It's not clear exactly how much of these asbestiform fibers are in our deodorants it's inclusion is not regulated in the manufacture of cosmetic products.

- *Silica* - Silica can act as a skin irritant, and as if that wasn't bad enough, there is also the chance that it could be contaminated with crystalline quartz, which is known to be a carcinogen. May also play a role in allergies and immunotoxicity.

So this is the situation – obviously we need deodorants in order to keep ourselves feeling and smelling fresh through the day, but many of the deodorants available in the store contain chemicals which can play a part in seriously damaging our health. The answer? Make safe deodorants at home using healthy, natural ingredients. They work like commercially bought deodorants, minus the dangers, and in addition, you'll also be able to save a little money and have fun! The process is simple, the ingredients are cheap, and many of the ingredients needed to make deodorants can be found in the average kitchen.

The All-Natural Ingredients You Can Use When Creating DIY Deodorants

One of the great things about creating your own deodorant is that you have total control over the ingredients you're going to use. In addition, gone are the days when sourcing hard to find ingredients seemed like an impossible task; nowadays, we can do a quick online search and find just about anything we want within a matter of seconds thanks to the power of almighty Google!

I admit that I wasn't exactly too crazy about making my own deodorant in the beginning. It seemed like it required too much effort. But all of that changed when I started doing my own research on the ingredients which could be used when making my own deodorant and began to understand the benefits each of these ingredients could have. I was so impressed that I had to try it out myself.

If you're feeling a bit overwhelmed by the idea of creating your own handmade deodorant, don't be. Once you get to know your ingredients better, you will be more than happy to make the transition.

Here are just some of the all-natural ingredients you can incorporate in making your own all-natural DIY deodorants.

- **Aloe Vera** - Aloe vera is packed with vitamins and minerals that don't just heal skin, they also lock in moisture. This gel-like substance is great for soothing and cooling skin. It's no wonder that Cleopatra is said to have used this miracle of nature as one of her go-to beauty regimen ingredients.

- ***Cocoa Butter*** - The same plant that gives us one of the best things ever, (chocolate!) also provides us with a skin softener like no other! Cocoa butter, which is rich in fatty acids, doesn't just smooth the skin, it can also do wonders in helping your skin stay soft and supple. A natural source of vitamin E, cocoa butter makes for the perfect moisturizer if used sparingly.

- ***Coconut Oil*** - One great thing about coconut oil is that it's safe to use on all skin types. Whether you're dealing with sensitive skin or you're one of the lucky ones who's blessed with problem-free skin, coconut oil makes a great all-around moisturizer. When used in deodorants, it helps keep the skin soft and free from microbes, fungi and other microorganisms.

- **_Lavender_** - This sweet-smelling flower, which is often used to treat anxiety and insomnia, also has a lesser-known beneficial property; the promotion of healthy cell turnover. As proof of its healing properties, ancient Romans used to wash injuries with lavender water. No wonder lavender is being touted as an herbal workhorse, helping to cure everything from hair loss to skin rashes!

- **_Olive Oil_** - We've all heard about the amazing effects this oil can have on the body when incorporated into a healthy diet. Olive oil is rich in antioxidants and vitamin E, which can help repair cell damage and fight free radicals. But olive oil isn't just great for skin care; it can also be a fantastic addition to your hair care routine.

Just apply a little onto a dry scalp, leave overnight, and you're guaranteed to wake up with healthier looking hair the next day. (For more on natural homemade shampoos, check out the book, "Homemade Shampoo: A Complete Beginner's Guide to Natural DIY Shampoos You Can Make Today", by me, Jane Aniston.)

- ***Shea butter*** - A superb moisturizer which has healing properties, making it a perfect ingredient for homemade deodorants. It is a rich source of Vitamins A and E, both of which help keep skin healthy and beautiful. Its fragrance is gentle and very soothing.

- ***Tea Tree Oil*** - You're probably well aware that tea tree oil is the number one natural acne fighter, but did you know that it's also one of the strongest all-natural antiseptics around? As an antibacterial agent, it acts like an all-purpose germ killer that can be used to treat anything from small insect bites to wounds. Some studies even show that it's more powerful than benzoyl peroxide in treating acne!

- ***Thyme*** - Has antibacterial and anti-fungal properties, making your all-natural deodorant a protective shield from the bacteria which cause the horrible sweaty smell!

- ***Apple cider vinegar*** - A substance which has numerous benefits, one of which is its antibacterial nature.

- ***Citrus fruit essential oils*** - When applied to the skin, citrus fruit oils can help neutralize unpleasant odors as well as increasing immunity against invading microorganisms.

- ***Mango butter*** - Great for treating dry skin and rejuvenating skin cells, leaving skin supple, smooth and young-looking.

- ***Bentonite clay*** - A substance known to eliminate toxins, impurities, chemicals and heavy metals from the body.

- ***Avocado butter*** - Rich in antioxidants, vitamins and minerals.

- ***Jasmine*** - Known to have anti-inflammatory and antiseptic benefits.

- ***Geranium*** - Non-irritating and can help promote circulation.

- ***Vetiver***- An essential oil extracted from the roots of Indian grass. Aside from its antiseptic qualities, vetiver can also help you relax. Vetiver's earthy fragrance is said to be effective in calming, stabilizing, balancing and soothing frayed nerves and emotions. This oil can also help dispel general pains.

- **_Cucumber_** - The list of cucumber's health benefits is really impressive! From its ability to hydrate skin, neutralize smells, supply the skin with vitamins and minerals, and its ability to flush out toxins, cucumber is an awesome ingredient!

With that said, we're almost ready to move on to the recipes, but before we do, I'll share with you my DIY deodorant insider secrets! Make sure you read through the next chapter carefully before moving on to the recipes. If you do you'll be well-prepared and ready to start on whipping up your first batch of chemical-free deodorant!

Chapter 2

Insider Tips On Creating Your Own Deodorants

It doesn't matter where you got your inspiration from, the important thing is that you've taken that first step to using much healthier, non-harmful deodorant. Making your own deodorants will be a lot of fun, but there are some things you should be aware of before you begin. So before you grab that mixing bowl, here are a few insider tips to get you off to a good start and help you avoid any problems further down the road.

Prep your workspace

The first thing you need to do before you get started on making your deodorants is to prep your workspace. Making your own deodorants at home can get quite messy, so make sure that you have prepared a dedicated space for it which will be easy to clean up when you've finished. Working in the kitchen is perfectly fine, but if you're going to turn it into a habit, you might want to look around your home for a small area you can dedicate to deodorant creation, space permitting of course.

Source your ingredients from a reliable supplier

Most of the ingredients needed to make your own homemade deodorants can easily be bought from grocery stores. However, if you're looking for an ingredient that can't be easily purchased in your area, you can always find a reliable supplier online with a little searching. When sourcing ingredients, make sure to choose a supplier that is known first and foremost for their quality, and not just the quantity of product they are offering. Don't be fooled by a cheap price tag if you're not sure about the quality of the product. Think of these ingredients as you would food; they will be entering your body through your skin, so chose the best you can find or that you can afford.

Be aware of your allergies

Just because an ingredient is considered all-natural or organic doesn't mean that it's guaranteed to be 100% safe for you. It may work wonders for others, but there is the odd chance that for you it could cause an allergic reaction. So before you get started on any homemade deodorants, make sure that the ingredients you're going to use are safe for you. Try to figure out which (if any) of the common ingredients may cause skin irritation. If you're going to work with an unfamiliar ingredient, test it first on your wrist to see if it causes a negative reaction. This way, you don't end up harming your skin in your quest for healthier deodorant alternatives.

Start with small batches

Since your homemade deodorant doesn't contain any chemical ingredients designed to prolong its lifespan, it's best to only make small batches at a time. Most of the recipes in this book will last for a matter of weeks, depending on the product. Therefore, it's highly recommended that you don't make too much at one time. However, as making fresh batches is quick, easy and fun, creating more is unlikely to be a major inconvenience.

Always store homemade deodorant in appropriate containers

Once you've made a fresh batch of DIY deodorant, it's critical that you store it in an appropriate container. As I mentioned above, your homemade deodorant won't contain any chemical preservatives to prevent bacterial growth, so always make it a point to use sterile containers. Look for containers with airtight lids so your product won't be exposed to air, humidity, germs, and bacteria. Although not essential, glass containers are a good option as glass is inert, meaning no chemicals will be able to leach into your deodorant.

Don't get too hung up on following the recipes to the letter

The amounts of the ingredients you'll need may seem a little vague (for example "1/8 cup" or "¼ teaspoon") but don't get too hung up on being exact; just follow the instructions as best you can to begin with. Making your own deodorants is a lot like cooking; over time you'll get used to the recipes and will be able to adjust them to suit your own needs and preferences.

Now that you're well prepared, let's get started on the recipes! Ive broken the recipes down into chapters based on type. Good luck!

Chapter 3

Fruity DIY Homemade Deodorant Recipes

These fruity DIY deodorants can keep you smelling sweet and fresh through the whole day. Unlike many store-bought deodorants though, the scents won't be too strong since the ingredients are all natural.

Here are five, affordable, easy-to-make, fruity deodorant recipes that even complete newbies can make with very little difficulty. Enjoy!

1. Sweet Orange & Thyme Homemade Deodorant

What do you get when you combine sweet orange and thyme, an aromatic plant from the mint family? Answer; a sweet, minty fragrance like no other! In addition, this deodorant will stop you from smelling without the risk of any negative side effects. Thyme has antibacterial and anti-fungal properties, making your all-natural deodorant a protective shield from harmful microorganisms. This recipe also contains apple cider vinegar, substance which has numerous medical benefits, one of which is its antibacterial nature. Although the production time may seem long (two weeks), the finished product is totally worth it!

Ingredients:

- The zest (the top layer of the orange's peel) of 1 orange

- ¼ cup fresh thyme

- ½ cup of apple cider vinegar

Instructions:

1. Put the thyme and the zest of orange in a container with a non-metallic lid.

2. Pour in the apple cider vinegar.

3. Let the mixture steep for 2 weeks. Make sure that you shake it for a few seconds occasionally (preferably everyday).

4. After two weeks, the deodorant is ready to use. Simply transfer the mixture into a spray bottle

and spray onto your underarms. Alternatively, pour one tablespoon of the deodorant over 2 cotton balls. Rub one cotton ball under each underarm.

Note: The recommended amount is good to last for 12-14 days if you use the deodorant once a day. Double the amount of each ingredient to have an adequate supply of this deodorant if you plan to use it more frequently. Make sure you don't make too much at one time (unless you are planning to give bottles away as gifts!) as this deodorant is best used within a month of production.

2. So Citrusy Non-Toxic Deodorant

The "so citrusy" fragrance of this deodorant makes it suitable for both men and women. When applied to the skin, citrus fruit oils can neutralize unpleasant odors and increase immunity against invading microorganisms. In addition, this recipe contains mango butter, bentonite clay, and carnauba wax. Mango butter is great for treating dry skin and in rejuvenating skin cells, making skin supple, smooth and young looking. On the other hand, bentonite clay is a substance known to eliminate toxins, impurities, chemicals and heavy metals from the body. What is carnauba wax? Well it's a popular nontoxic and hypoallergenic ingredient used in some food and cosmetic products.

Ingredients:

- 5 tablespoons mango butter

- 10 drops of each of the following essential oils:

    - Lemon

    - Lemon grass

    - Grapefruit

    - Tangerine

- 2 tablespoons carnauba wax (easily available online if you can't find it locally)

- 2 tablespoons bentonite clay

Instructions:

1. Clean used deodorant sticks holders thoroughly. Ensure that all traces of the store

bought deodorants are gone. Set aside to dry. Another option is to simply use small sterile pots, but then you'll have to apply the deodorant with your fingers.

2. In a small saucepan, pour the carnauba wax and mango butter. Set over a low flame.

3. Stir the ingredients until fully melted. It should become a gooey paste. Place into a glass bowl.

4. Allow the paste to cool slightly.

5. Add the benotine clay to the paste, along with the essential oils and stir gently until mixed.

6. Pour the warm finished product into the used deodorant sticks or sterile pots. This recipe should last for 2-3 months, depending on how often you use the deodorant.

Note: Another version of this recipe is to use avocado butter instead of mango butter. Avocado butter is rich in antioxidants, vitamins and minerals. In addition, it can lighten skin tone, hydrate and nourish the skin and help prevent breakouts.

Also, if some of the essential oils are not available, you can replace them with pomelo or orange oils. It will still give you that "so citrusy" fragrance.

3. DIY All-Natural Citrus Spray Deodorant

Through the years, citrus fruits have been proven effective in keeping skin looking healthy, smooth and beautiful. Plus, their smell is undeniably refreshing and invigorating. This recipe includes four different citrus fruits plus Melissa water (which you'll be able to find online). This super- simple recipe is so easy that even a complete novice should be able to complete the procedure in a matter of minutes.

Ingredients

- 3 ½ tablespoons of each of the following ingredients:

- Orange peel

- Witch hazel

- Lemon water

- Melissa water

- 10 drops of lemon essential oil

- 20 drops of:

  - Tangerine essential oil

  - Sweet orange essential oil

Instructions

1. Place the first four ingredients in a jug.

2. Add the three essential oils.

3. Mix well.

4. Use a funnel and transfer this mixture into a spray bottle.

5. That's it. You have a spray deodorant that you can spray directly onto your armpits anytime.

Note: For variation, you can try other combinations of citrus essential oils. Mix and match these oils until you achieve the combination that you really like. Make sure to jot down your personalized deodorant recipes when you find one which you really like.

4. Cool Lemon DIY Deodorant

When life gives you lemons, make deodorant out of them! With this recipe you will be able to enjoy the freshness and coolness that lemons can bring to your underarms. This recipe also contains coconut oil, arrowroot, and baking soda. Arrowroot is an herb that contains starch, and in combination with the baking soda, helps keep underarms dry without clogging the sweat glands. The extra virgin coconut oil has numerous medical properties and has been used for centuries. When used in deodorants, it helps make the skin soft and keep it free from microbes, fungi and other microorganisms.

Ingredients

- 10 drops lemon essential oil

- 2 tablespoons of baking soda

- 2 tablespoons arrowroot

- 1 tablespoon extra virgin coconut oil

Instructions

1. Mix the baking soda and arrowroot thoroughly in a small bowl.

2. Pour in the extra virgin coconut oil and the lemon essential oil. Mix well.

3. Place the finished product into used deodorant containers or sterile pots.

4. Place the mixture in the refrigerator for 30 minutes (or until it solidifies). At this time, the deodorant is ready to use.

Note: If you live somewhere where the climate is temperate, keep these deodorants in the refrigerator, as coconut oil will melt at temperatures of 76 degrees fahrenheit and higher.

If you'd prefer not to use baking soda, simply replace it with GMO-free cornstarch.

5. 3-in-1 All-Natural Homemade Deodorants

This amazing deodorant recipe is a combination of herbs, flowers and citrus oils. The finished product is a gentle deodorant with antibacterial properties which can be used by both men and women. A little vodka is used in this recipe and acts as a preservative.

Ingredients:

- The citrus fruit essential oils are:

  - 10 drops bergamot oil

  - 5 drops of lemon oil

  - 2 drops of mandarin oil

- The herb essential oils are:

    - 7 drops of thyme oil

    - 8 drops of Clary sage oil

    - 5 drops of rosewood oil

    - 3 drops of lavender oil

- The flower waters are:

    - 4 tablespoons of witch hazel

    - 2 tablespoons of orange flower water

    - 2 tablespoons of linden flower water

- 1 teaspoon of vodka

Instructions

1. Pour the vodka in a clean, 4 oz. spray bottle (preferably made of glass).

2.   Add the essential oils carefully one at a time.

3.   Shake very well to dissolve the oils.

4.   Pour the witch hazel into the bottle.

5.   Next, pour the remaining 2 flower waters.

6.   Shake well each time before use.

Note: Vodka is a neutral spirit made from the distillation of wheat, rye, potatoes, fruits, sugars and other foods that can be fermented. Don't worry, when combined with the other ingredients the smell of the vodka will be completely hidden.

Chapter 4

Green and Easy Vegan DIY Deodorant Recipes

Green is in – not only for our diets but also for skin care and beauty products. No one can deny the health benefits of going green. Hence, more and more people are turning to vegetables and herbs for their meals, drinks, and now, even for their deodorants.

In this chapter, there are four amazing deodorant recipes that make use of various vegetables and herbs that can be bought at any grocery store. If you'd like a steady supply of herbs, why not have a small container garden in your kitchen if you have the space? This way you'll be sure that there are no pesticides or other chemicals used to produce them.

Either way, here are four easy and healthy vegan DIY deodorant recipes. Enjoy!

6. Aloe Vera Wonder Deodorant

Considered as one of nature's best cleansers, aloe vera is the perfect choice to use as an ingredient for your homemade deodorant. In this recipe, we'll be using the gel of the aloe vera. This is the clear, jelly-like substance located in the inner part of the aloe leaves. This recipe is affordable, easy and highly effective in keeping underarms dry and fresh all day long!

Ingredients

- 1 tablespoon olive oil

- 1 tablespoon of vegetable glycerin

- 2 tablespoons of aloe vera gel

- 4 tablespoons baking soda

- 10 drops of any essential oil of your choice

Instructions

1. Over a medium heat, place a saucepan with all the ingredients in it except for the essential oil.

2. Gently stir with a spoon until the ingredients are thoroughly mixed.

3. Add the essential oils and stir them into the mixture.

4. Store in sterile pots and apply to the underarms as needed.

Note: Try combining different essential oils to give your aloe deodorant a unique scent of your own!

7. Mix and Match Aromatic Herbal Deodorant

The beauty of this recipe is its versatility. In this recipe, dried or fresh sage is recommended, but you can actually use other aromatic herbs that you like, for instance thyme or rosewood. At the same time, you can also substitute in your favorite essential oils. Be creative and discover a whole new world of aromatic herbal deodorants. This recipe requires some time and efforts but the end result is well worth it!

Ingredients

- ¼ cup of dried or fresh garden sage (if fresh herbs are used, you'll need to mince them)

- ¼ cup of dried or fresh sage

- ¼ cups of dried or fresh lavender flower

- ½ cup of lemon rind, sliced (organic is preferable)

- 1 tablespoon vodka (80 proof recommended)

- Essential oils (not needed until the second stage of production)

    - 30 drops lavender

    - 30 drops lemon

    - 15 drops sage

- ½ teaspoon of vegetable glycerin (optional)

Instructions

1. If using fresh ingredients, make sure that they are minced well before starting on the recipe.

2. Place the fresh or dried ingredients in a jar. Toss the sliced lemon rinds into the jar on top.

3. Pour the vodka on top of the ingredients in the jar. Cap the jar tightly. (Note: Do not add the essential oils at this point!)

4. Let it sit for 4 weeks, making sure that you shake it for a few seconds each day.

5. After the allotted time has passed, strain the herbs.

6. Filter the concoction through a fine mesh strainer into a clean mason jar. Squeeze the herbs as you filter.

7. Add the glycerin plus all the essential oils.

8. Replace the cap tightly. Shake vigorously for 30 seconds.

9. Using a funnel, transfer the contents into spray bottles.

10. Cap. Label properly. Store in a cool, dry and dark place.

Note: Before using the deodorant, shake the bottle well. Spray onto clean, dry underarms. Allow to dry before you put on your clothing. Alternatively you can also pour a tablespoon of the liquid deodorant onto 2 cotton balls or pads and swab onto the underarms.

8. Cool And Clean Cucumber Deodorant

The list of cucumber's health benefits is really impressive! From its ability to hydrate skin, neutralize smells, supply the skin with vitamins and minerals, and its ability to flush out toxins, cucumber is an awesome ingredient! Add lavender or juniper scents to make this fantastic deodorant.

Ingredients

- 15 drops of lavender or juniper essential oil (whichever you prefer)

- 2 tablespoons aloe vera juice

- 2 tablespoons of organic cucumber juice

- 1 tablespoon of baking soda

- ½ teaspoon vodka

Instructions

1. Put the baking soda in a clean spray bottle.

2. Pour in the cucumber and aloe vera juices.

3. Add the vodka.

4. Pour the essential oils. Shake gently for 30 seconds.

That's it! You can spritz it directly onto your clean underarms or pour it onto cotton balls and swab onto your underarms.

Note: Cucumber is affordable, readily available and useful in eliminating toxins from the body, too. Try to add cucumber to your water or consume it raw regularly to help your body remove toxins.

9. Herbal Power DIY Deodorant

This deodorant has a great musky scent which is great for men. The witch hazel in this recipe adds a cleanness to the scent. The recipe is effortless, very cheap, non-irritating, and effective in fighting off body odor.

Ingredients

- ½ cup of pure distilled water

- 1 tablespoon of witch hazel

- 3 drops of juniper essential oil

- 10 drops of cedar wood essential oil

Instructions

1. In a clean container or spray bottle, combine the distilled water and witch hazel.

2. Add in the essential oils.

3. Stir or shake gently.

4. Store in a cool, dry place.

Note: As with other spray deodorants, shake well before using. If you are feeling adventurous, you can add other essential oils to create a new scent while maintaining the masculine scent. Example is coriander essential oil, which also possesses a musky, woody and spicy scent, ideal for men.

Chapter 5

Flower Power All Natural DIY Deodorant Recipes

Flowers have always been popular when it comes to skin care and beauty products, which is not surprising considering that flowers not only possess fragrant scents, most of them also possess medicinal properties. For instance, jasmine is known for its anti-inflammatory and antiseptic benefits. Hops flowers are astringent, antimicrobial, antiseptic and bactericidal. Lavender is commonly used for its fresh smell but in addition has lesser known antimicrobial and anti-inflammatory properties. Geranium is non-irritating plus it promotes circulation. It makes the skin healthier and softer, too. Ylang ylang is not commonly seen except in tropical countries. It has a very sweet smell. It is effective against bacteria and other harmful organisms.

In this chapter we'll cover a number of wonderful deodorant recipes that use flowers as their main ingredient.

10. Lavender Wonder DIY All Natural Deodorant

Try this easy-to-make recipe which includes sweet, musky, citrus and minty scents, the combination of which is truly wonderful!

Ingredients

- 3 ½ tablespoons of lavender water

- 7 tablespoons of rose water

- 3 ½ tablespoons of geranium water

- 20 drops of lavender essential oil

- 10 drops of lemon essential oil

- 20 drops of geranium essential oil

Instructions

1. Pour all of the flower waters into a clean jar or jug.

2. Add the essential oils one at a time.

3. Mix well

4. Using a funnel, transfer the concoction into a spray bottle (preferably glass).

5. Shake before using. Spritz onto the armpit as necessary.

11. Fresh Jasmine Delight Homemade Deodorant

You'll be delighted with this divine concoction of coconut oil and Jasmine essential oil. Jasmine is ideal for everyday use and it's calming, relaxing and rich smell can soothe the nerves.

Ingredients

- 1 tablespoon jasmine essential oil

- 5 tablespoons coconut oil

- 3 tablespoons cornstarch

- 3 tablespoons baking soda

Instructions

1. In a dry bowl, combine the baking soda and cornstarch.

2. Add the coconut oil and stir until well blended (if the coconut oil is in a solid state, heat gently until liquid). There should be no lumps.

3. Pour in the jasmine essential oil and mix gently.

4. Place in the refrigerator for several minutes until the oil begins to solidify.

5. Transfer into a clean container with a lid.

6. During summer, you can keep the deodorant in the refrigerator to maintain its solid state, although when it is melted it can be easier to apply. Simply scoop a little of the deodorant out and rub onto clean underarms.

Note: This deodorant could last up to 2-3 months. If you sweat or perspire profusely, you can add an additional 2 teaspoons of both arrowroot powder the baking soda. Take note though that some people react to baking soda and they complain of skin irritation. If in doubt test a little of the deodorant on a small patch of skin before use. If you'd prefer not to us baking soda try replacing it with   arrowroot powder in equal measure.

12. 5 Flower Cypress Deodorant

A sublime combination of sweet floral scents from five flowers and the fine woody scent of cypress! Add a hint of citrus and voila; you have a delightfully unique aroma that you won't find among commercially prepared deodorants. This wonderful fragrance is suitable for both men and women. It also makes a great gift for friends and family members. Try it today!

Ingredients

- Essential oils:

    10 drops of geranium

    4 drops of lavender

5 drops of neroli

10 drops of cypress

8 drops of bergamot

3 drops of black pepper

- 4 tablespoons of witch hazel

- 2 tablespoons of orange flower water

- 2 tablespoons of cornflower water

- 1 teaspoon of high proof vodka

Instructions

1. Pour the vodka into a spray bottle (preferably glass). Add the essential oils one at a time.

2. Shake the bottle vigorously to disperse and dissolve the essential oils.

3. Pour the witch hazel into the bottle.

4. Add the two remaining flower waters. Shake well.

5. Label the bottle and the deodorant is ready to be used anytime!

Note: Remember to shake the bottle very well before spraying onto clean underarms.

Chapter 6

Non-Toxic Oil and Butter Deodorant Recipes

Coconut oil contains fatty acids and numerous powerful medicinal properties. It has been proven to stave off viruses, bacteria, fungi and other harmful pathogens. It is also a popular choice of ingredient in various skin care and beauty products because of its ability to moisturize the skin deeply.

Butters, on the other hand, are also popular when it comes to helping keep skin beautiful, soft and supple. Just like coconut oil, many body butters have medicinal properties that can protect the skin from damage and premature aging.

When you combine coconut oil (and other healthy oils) along with body butters, you have the perfect combination for a skin-care product, and specifically for deodorants. As an alternative to store-bought deodorants, you simply can't go wrong with natural oils and butters as the base ingredients for your homemade deodorants.

In this chapter we have some super-soothing and highly effective deodorant recipes using the aforementioned butters and oils. Although there are no reports of clothes being stained by the ingredients in these recipes, due to the nature of oils and butters it's still advised to allow these deodorants to be absorbed by the skin and for the underarms to feel dry to the touch before getting dressed. Use sparingly and use caution with your clothing if you have any concerns.

13. Virgin Coconut Oil & Shea Butter DIY Deodorant

Shea butter is a superb moisturizer which has healing properties, making it a perfect ingredient for homemade deodorants. It is a rich source of Vitamins A and E, both of which help keep skin healthy and beautiful. Its fragrance is gentle and very soothing.

Ingredients

- 2 tablespoons of Shea butter

- 3 tablespoons of virgin coconut oil

- 3 tablespoons of baking soda

- 2 tablespoons of cornstarch

- 5 drops of essential oil (your pick)

Instructions

1. In a small pan or preferably a double boiler, allow the coconut oil and Shea butter to melt together on low heat. Turn off the heat when this is achieved.

2. Add the baking soda and cornstarch. Stir thoroughly until the mixture is completely smooth. There should be no lumps.

3. Add the essential oil. Allow it to cool.

4. Place in a clean container.

Note: It's recommended you use a double boiler because the butter and oil tend to burn easily. If you do not have a double boiler, you can improvise using a saucepan and a mixing bowl (made of glass/pyrex or metal). Make sure that the two items fit together snugly. There should be no gap between the bowl and the saucepan because you need the steam of the simmering water in the saucepan to heat the bowl which in turn will melt the oils.

Add water to the pan, bring it to a gentle simmer and then place the bowl on top. The bowl should not touch the water in the pan. Melt the butter and oil in the mixing bowl, then follow the rest of the steps in the process.

Another method in the absence of double boiler (and this is a useful method if you are just making a small amount of deodorant) is directly using a small glass mason jar. Just place the oil and butter inside the jar and place the jar in a small saucepan of simmering water until the oil and butter melt. Then simply follow the rest of the instructions, leaving out number 4, as the container that you'll make the deodorant in is the one you can use for it's storage.

When using the deodorant, simply scoop a small amount in your hand and then rub onto clean underarms. During summer or if you live in a warm country, place the deodorant inside the refrigerator to solidify the coconut oil.

14. 3-Ingredient DIY Homemade Deodorant

If you'd prefer to stick to the basics, the two following "3- ingredients" recipes might be the answer. These recipes don't contain any essential oils and consequently are almost odorless, meaning not only are these recipes effective at keeping you sweat-free, they're also perfect for those who aren't so keen on strong scents.

Ingredients

- 3 tablespoons coconut oil

- 3 tablespoons baking soda

- 2 tablespoons Shea butter

Instructions

1. Melt the coconut oil and Shea butter in a double boiler (or in an improvised double boiler as detailed at the end of the previous recipe).

2. Remove from heat. Add the baking soda.

3. Mix well and leave to cool and your deodorant is ready for use.

Note: You can add arrowroot (2 tablespoons) to this recipe (at the same time as you add the baking soda) to make it even more effective at controlling perspiration. In addition, if you'd like this deodorant to be scented, add 5-10 drops of any essential oils that you like after adding the baking soda. Experiment until you discover the perfect combination of oils for

the scent you like.

15. Super-Simple 3-Ingredient Deodorant

If you thought the 3-ingredients DIY Homemade deodorant in the last recipe was simple enough, you may be surprised to find out the recipe can be made even simpler! In this recipe we can do away with the Shea butter and the double boiler making the recipe perfect if you are too busy to make one of the more complicated concoctions!

Ingredients

- 6 tablespoons of coconut oil

- 4 tablespoons of baking soda

- 4 tablespoons of cornstarch (or arrowroot powder if you prefer)

Instructions

1. Mix the baking soda and cornstarch together in a bowl.

2. Mash the coconut oil into the mixture until the ingredients are well combined.

3. Stir very well until smooth.

4. Place in a clean container.

Note: What could be simpler and easier than that, right? This recipe may well be the best of all in terms of time required, simplicity of preparation and value for money.

Chapter 7

Mix & Match Ingredient Natural DIY Deodorants

The deodorant recipes in the previous chapters were categorized according to their main ingredient. In this chapter however, we'll be mixing and matching the ingredients, so if you can't decide which type of recipe in this book sounds most appealing, why not try out one of these fantastic mix and match combination recipes!

Some ingredients here may come as a bit of a surprise and some may sound unfamiliar; for instance vetiver and food grade diatomaceous earth. Don't worry though; these ingredients are readily available online if you decide you'd like to give these recipes a go.

Here are five recipes that combine a range of different ingredients to form uniquely wonderful DIY deodorants. In addition, there are DIY deodorant recipes included here which will be of particular interest to those who have either extra sensitive skin or super sweaty underarms.

16. Organic Butter, Oil, Fruit, Herb, Flower Combo All-Natural Deodorant

A fantastic deodorant which uses a wide range of ingredients and has a wonderful fragrance that's hard to describe.

Ingredients

- 1/8 cup of organic cocoa butter

- 1/8 cup of Shea butter

- ½ tablespoon of baking soda

- 1/8 cup of organic arrowroot powder

- 5 drops of Vitamin E oil

- 5-10 drops of the following (organic) essential oils

    - Fir Needle

- Grapefruit

- Nutmeg

- Lavender

Instructions

1. Combine the Shea butter and cocoa butter in a mixing bowl (pyrex or metal preferable).

2. In a double boiler, (see Virgin Coconut Oil & Shea Butter DIY Deodorant recipe for a simple method of improvising a double boiler) melt the butters over a low-medium heat.

3. Remove from heat when the butters are melted. Add in the baking soda and arrowroot powder. Stir the mixture gently.

4. Pour in the Vitamin E oil and the essential oils. (If you prefer simply take a vitamin E capsule, carefully prick with a pin and squeeze 5 drops into the mixture).

5. Stir gently until the ingredients are combined.

6. Place into clean containers. Cover lightly with a lid (so that dust will not settle on the mixture) and let it set.

7. When the deodorant has completely cooled and is in a solid state (which can take up to 6 hours), cap tightly and store in a dry, cool place.

Note: This recipe will give you 2 ounces of deodorant, which should last for around 2 weeks depending on how much you use.

17. Vetiver And Orange Spray Deodorant

So what is vetiver? It is an essential oil extracted from the roots of Indian grass, and luckily it can easily be purchased online! Aside from its antiseptic qualities, vetiver can also help you relax. Vetiver's earthy fragrance is said to be effective in calming, stabilizing, balancing and soothing frayed nerves and emotions. General pains can also be dispelled with the use of this oil. The orange essential oil adds to the therapeutic effects of the vetiver.

Ingredients

- 2 tablespoons of witch hazel

- 3 drops vetiver essential oil

- 10 drops orange essential oil

Instructions

1. Pour the witch hazel in a clean container.

2. Add the essential oils one after the other.

3. Mix well.

4. Transfer to a clean spray bottle (preferably glass) and store in a cool, dry place.

Note: There are many variations of this recipe. Adding several essential oils can totally change the fragrance without negating its effects. The only thing I'd recommend is that you keep the amount of vetiver and orange higher than any other essential oils that you decide to add.

18. Oil, Butter, Clay, & Tea Tree Surprise DIY Deodorant

Tea tree is antibacterial, anti-fungal, antiseptic plus it's hypoallergenic. It's very popular as a skin and beauty product ingredient for its many known uses and therapeutic effects.

Ingredients

- 2 cups extra virgin coconut oil

- 25 drops of tea tree essential oil

- 1 ½ tablespoons of beeswax beads or shavings

- ¾ cup of arrowroot powder

- ¼ cup of baking soda

- 5 drops of lemongrass essential oil

- 2 tablespoons bentonite clay

Instructions

1. Using a double boiler, (see Virgin Coconut Oil & Shea Butter DIY Deodorant recipe for a simple method of improvising a double boiler) place the coconut oil and beeswax on a low heat and when it is barely melted, remove it from the heat.

2. Add the rest of the ingredients one at a time except for the essential oils.

3. While allowing the mixture to cool, stir continuously.

4. The mixture will reach a pudding-like consistency. At this point, add the essential oils and mix thoroughly.

5. Transfer into clean containers.

6. Leave overnight to harden before use.

Note: This recipe can fill up to three containers (depending on the size) and can last up to a month (depending on usage).

19. Anti Super-Sweaty Armpits Deodorants

Some unlucky people suffer from overly-active sweat glands, causing them to perspire profusely. The hassle of having wet underarms can be extremely irritating and can also cause feelings of self-consciousness. Luckily, this homemade deodorant can help tackle excessive sweating without the need for any nasty chemicals. The food grade diatomaceous earth (which you can easily purchase online) is a substance that many people are not aware of but which really adds to this recipe.

Ingredients

- 30 grams coconut oil

- 20 grams Shea butter

- 10 grams beeswax

- 10 grams almond oil (or other oil that you prefer)

- 15 grams arrowroot powder

- 5 drops of vitamin E

- 15 grams food grade diatomaceous earth

- 20-25 drops of any essential oils (if you would like to use a variety of essential oils, simply make sure that the total number of drops is between 20-25)

Instructions

1. Using a double boiler (see Virgin Coconut Oil & Shea Butter DIY Deodorant recipe for a simple method of improvising a double boiler) set over low heat, place the Shea butter, oils and beeswax

to melt. Stir gently until everything has melted. The last thing to melt should be the beeswax.

2. When fully melted, remove from heat. Set aside and allow to cool for a while.

3. Add the arrowroot, vitamin E and food grade diatomaceous earth. Whisk vigorously.

4. Add the essential oil. If you choose more than one essential oil, add them one at a time. Then mix well.

5. Pour into clean containers and allow to set. This should take around 30 minutes or less. When set, your anti super-sweaty deodorant is ready for use.

Note: Beeswax is made from the wax secreted by bees. It has a wide variety of uses. However, a very small number of people are allergic to beeswax. If you are allergic to beeswax, you can replace it with carnauba wax. For the vegans, soy wax is another alternative.

20. DIY All Natural Deodorant For Sensitive Skin

The chicken or the egg conundrum can also apply to caring for sensitive skin; do harsh cosmetics cause sensitive skin, or was the skin always susceptible to irritants? Whatever the truth, a simple solution is to use all natural, organic (as much as possible), and fresh ingredients in all products that will touch our skin. In this recipe, only basic ingredients are used to ensure dry underarms without skin irritation.

Ingredients

- ¾ cup organic arrowroot powder (a good substitute is non-GMO cornstarch)

- ¼ cup of baking soda

- 6 tablespoons of melted coconut oil

Instructions

1. In a bowl, combine the arrowroot powder and baking soda.

2. Add the melted coconut oil and stir in using a fork. Mix until there are no more lumps.

3. Transfer the mixture into a clean container and cap tightly.

Note: If you are not satisfied with the consistency of the finished product, add more coconut oil. Continue to stir until you reach the desired consistency. To use, just scoop out a small amount and apply to clean underarms.

For those who are unfortunate enough that even this gentle recipe irritates their sensitive skin, one option is to simply try melted coconut oil alone which can act as a very basic deodorant.

Conclusion

The way we choose to spend our money is important. If we continue to support companies that make a profit from endangering our health, it could be said that we are exercising poor judgment and failing to act wisely.

I believe it's important that we each do our own research into the deodorants we buy and use. For our health's sake, as well as the health of others who use these products, it pays to be an informed consumer and to vote with our dollars.

Thank you again for downloading this book. I hope you enjoyed reading it and were able to learn a lot about the benefits of making your own deodorant at home. What's more, I hope you will actually try some of the recipes for yourself and that you're able to experience the benefits of using these natural, healthy alternatives to store-bought deodorants!

A message from the author, Jane Aniston

Finally, if you enjoyed this book, **please** take the time to post a review on Amazon. It will only take a couple of minutes and I'd be extremely grateful for your support.

Jane Aniston

FREE BONUS!: Preview Of "Homemade Makeup - A Complete Beginner's Guide to Natural DIY Cosmetics You Can Make Today" - Includes 28 Organic Makeup Recipes!'

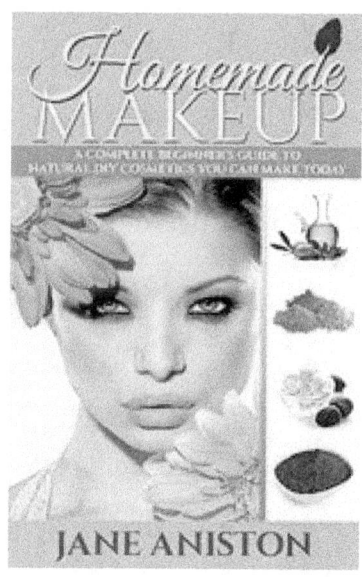

If you enjoyed this book, I have a little bonus for you; a preview of one of my other books "Homemade Makeup - A Complete Beginner's Guide to Natural DIY Cosmetics You Can Make Today", which exposes the secrets of the hidden toxins lurking in your store-bought cosmetics! This book also includes 28 simple and enjoyable organic makeup recipes that you can make at home today. Give yourself a glamorous look without exposing yourself to potentially harmful chemical nasties! Enjoy!

Chapter 1: Why you should stop using store-bought makeup and start making your own at home!

Makeup is something most women simply can't live without. Some women, in their search for beauty, have even gone as far getting permanent cosmetics tattooed on their faces (permanent eyebrows, for example). Personally, I see nothing wrong with wanting to look your best, but at the end of the day, one question we need to ask ourselves is: "What exactly are the ingredients in my beauty products?"

With almost all cosmetics containing numerous chemical ingredients, it can be a bit unsettling to think about the potential long-term effects these ingredients could be having on our bodies. Behind the glamour of the cosmetics industry, there's always the danger that the products we think are safe to put on our skin, might in actuality not be as safe as we think.

After studying the cosmetics industry, the truth is that these products have some of the largest mark-ups of any you're likely to find on the high street or in the mall! Your favorite face cream that cost you $80 may well have only cost as little as $2 to make, while that trendy lipstick you paid $30 of your hard-earned money for may actually only have a monetary value of $0.75! If you've bought thousands of dollars worth of cosmetics over the years, this realization can be pretty depressing. It doesn't feel good to know that all this time we've been duped by the cosmetics industry via slick marketing campaigns, while they made massive profits out of us unsuspecting consumers.

This is certainly something I've been a victim of. In the past, one of the things I would regularly spend money on was a good (and very expensive!) lipstick. Whenever I was having a bad day, I would head down to my favorite store and treat myself to a new shade. My friends would easily be able to tell if I was having a good year or not by the number of lipsticks I had in my collection! In hindsight, knowing what I know now, I feel a real sense of regret that I didn't get around to making my own cosmetics earlier. If I had of done, my bank balance certainly would have been a little healthier, and that money could have been better put to use.

The thing about the cosmetics industry is that even if you have a suspicion you're being ripped-off, it just feels that buying these products is something you *have to do*. I know a lot of women who would gladly fork over an inordinate amount of money for an excellent foundation! Why? Because you simply can't put a price on the confidence that looking your best can give you. The marketing used to sell cosmetic products has preyed on the insecurities of women for far too long. We are constantly bombarded with the message that if you want to feel good about yourself you need to look like a cover model; the implication being that the only way you'll be able to do that is to use their (expensive!) cosmetics. It's even gotten to the point where some women consider certain brands of makeup to be status symbols, much like they may do with a pair of expensive shoes or a designer handbag.

Am I immune to the marketing hype surrounding cosmetics? Honestly, no. I confess that even after learning the heartbreaking truth about the beauty industry I still get excited when I'm in the store browsing the makeup department. I still look at each lipstick color and eye shadow shade and imagine how I would incorporate them to achieve all sorts of glamorous looks. The only difference now is I don't purchase anywhere near as many products as I used to. These days I usually just look around in search of color inspiration, make a mental note and then create my own cosmetics at home. If you're thinking that the only reason I do this is to save a few dollars, you're wrong. Unfortunately there's more to it than that.

Harmful Ingredients Abound!

One of the sad realities when it comes to cosmetics is that the vast majority contain toxic ingredients. Even makeup products labeled as "all-natural" often times contain ingredients that may increase susceptibility to skin allergies, cancer, infertility and reproductive problems. If you're not sure about which ingredients you'd be best to avoid, here's a list of chemical nasties which are often used in cosmetics. Considering that human skin absorbs almost 60% of what is applied to it, this list will make you think twice next time you're about to splurge on expensive cosmetics.

- **Coal Tar** – Although already banned in the EU and Southeast Asia, there are still some products being sold in the US that contain this carcinogen. It's often found in treatments for dry skin as well as in anti-dandruff shampoos. Coal tar is also known as FD&C Red No.6.

- **Ethoxylated surfactants and 1,4-dioxane** – Created when carcinogenic ethylene oxide is added to a cocktail of other chemicals. This nasty toxin is found in some cosmetics, and unfortunately, is commonly found in baby washes being sold in the US. As a general rule, if you want to err on the safe side, avoid ingredients that contain the syllable "eth".

- **Fragrance/"Parfum"** – A catchall for unknown chemicals like phthalates. Fragrance has been proven to cause dizziness, headaches, asthma, and even allergic reactions in some unsuspecting victims.

- **Formaldehyde** – A proven irritant and likely carcinogen that can be found in hair dye, nail products, and shampoos. It is already banned in the EU.

- **Lead** – A carcinogenic contaminant found in most lipsticks and hair dyes. Since it's not officially considered to be an ingredient, you'll never see this listed on any beauty product.

- **Hydroquinone** – An ingredient used to peal and lighten skin. It is banned in the UK due to the fact it's been linked to cancer and reproductive disorders.

- **Mineral oil** – This petroleum byproduct can be found in moisturizers, baby oils, and styling gels.

- **Mercury** – An allergen that is known to impair brain function and development. Can be found in select eye drops and mascaras.

- **Parabens** – Used to preserve ingredients in many beauty and baby products. Has been linked to cancer, reproductive disorders, and endocrine problems.

- **Oxybenzone** – A chemical sunscreen that accumulates in fat cells. It can cause allergic reactions and hormone irregularity.

- **Phthalates** – A type of plasticizer that is banned in the EU and just recently, in California. It can be found in perfumes, deodorants, and lotions; and has been linked to kidney, liver, and lung damage.

- **Paraphenylenediamine (PPD)** – Present in hair dyes and styling products. Proven to be toxic to skin and can cause complications with the immune system.

- **Silicone derived emollients** – An ingredient added to some cosmetic products to make them feel soft. It has been linked to skin irritation and tumor enlargement.

- **Talc** – Has a similar composition to asbestos. Can be found in some blushes, eye shadows, baby powders, and deodorants. Has been linked to respiratory problems and ovarian cancer.

- **Sodium lauryl (ether) sulphate (SLS, SLES)** – An ingredient added to soap to make it foamy. It's easily absorbed by the body and can lead to irritation of sensitive skin.

- **Triclosan** – Can be found in some hand sanitizers, deodorants, and antibacterial products. It has been linked to endocrine disorders and cancer.

- **Toluene** – Has been linked to endocrine and immune disorders. Often found in hair and nail products, this ingredient is often hidden under the term, "fragrance."

Check out the rest of "Homemade Makeup: A Complete Beginner's Guide To Natural DIY Cosmetics You Can Make Today" by Jane Aniston on Amazon.

Check Out My Other Books!

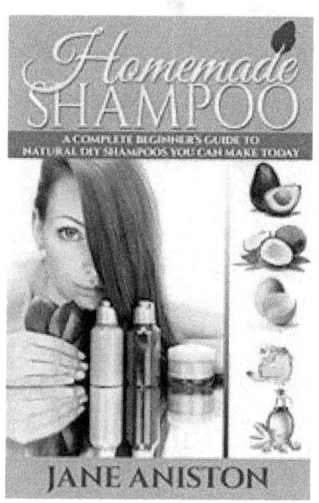

Homemade Shampoo (Includes 34 Organic Shampoo Recipes!)

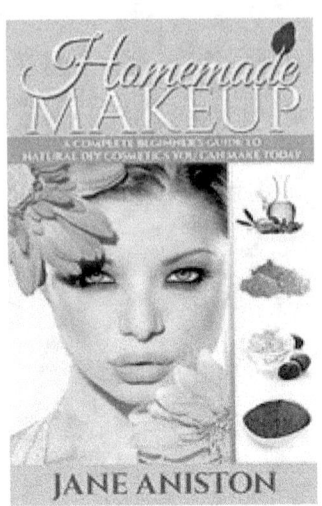

Homemade Makeup (Includes 28 Organic Makeup Recipes!)

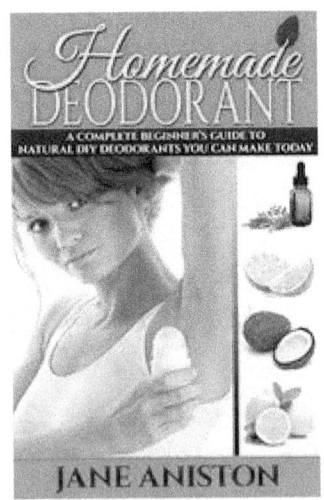

Homemade Deodorant (Includes 20 Organic Deodorant Recipes!)

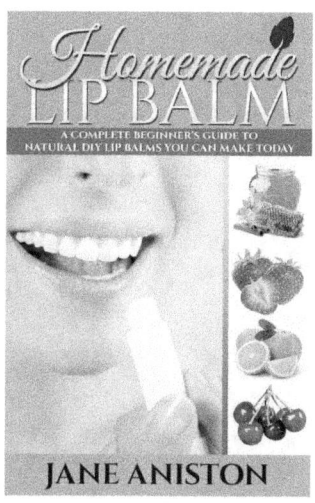

Homemade Lip Balm (Includes 22 Organic Lip Balm Recipes!)

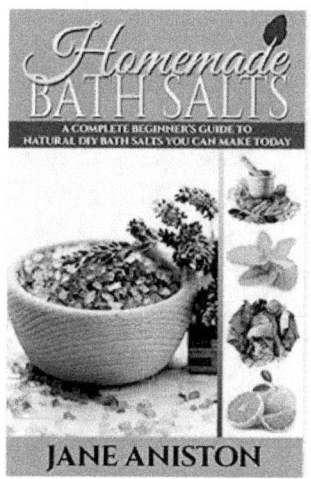

Homemade Bath Salts (Includes 35 Organic Bath Salt Recipes!)